DR. BARBARA'S MUCUS CLEANSE DIET

Revitalize your health:discover dr.Barbara's mucus cleanse diet- a proven path to detoxify, energies and achieve optimal well-bell naturally

Ben Hans

Table of Contents

COPYRIGHT © 2023

CHAPTER ONE

Introduction to the Mucus Cleanse Diet

The Mucus Cleanse Diet, also known as the Mucusless Diet, has gained popularity in recent years as a natural approach to detoxification and improving overall health. This dietary regimen is based on the principles outlined by Arnold Ehret, a German health educator and advocate for naturopathy in the early 20th century. Ehret proposed that excessive mucus accumulation in the body was the root cause of various ailments and diseases, and thus advocated for a diet aimed at eliminating mucus-forming foods.

Historical Context

To understand the Mucus Cleanse Diet, it's essential to delve into its historical context. Arnold Ehret, born in 1866, was influenced by the naturopathic movement of his time, which emphasized natural healing methods and lifestyle interventions. Ehret himself suffered from health issues during his youth, which led him to explore alternative approaches to wellness. Through his own experiences and observations, he developed his theories on the relationship between diet, mucus formation, and disease.

Ehret's ideas were largely shaped by his study of physiology and the works of other health reformers of his time, such as Sylvester Graham and John H. Tilden. He believed that the modern diet, characterized by excessive consumption of meat, dairy, refined grains, and processed foods, contributed to the accumulation of mucus in the body, leading to a host of health problems.

Principles of the Mucus Cleanse Diet

Central to the Mucus Cleanse Diet is the classification of foods into two categories: mucus-forming and mucusless. According to Ehret, mucus-forming foods are those that leave behind a residue of mucus in the body after digestion, while mucusless foods are those that do not produce such residue. The goal of the diet is to minimize or eliminate mucus-forming foods while emphasizing mucusless foods to promote detoxification and healing.

Mucus-forming foods include animal products such as meat, dairy, and eggs, as well as refined grains, processed foods, and certain fruits and vegetables, particularly those that are high in starch or sugar. In contrast, mucusless foods consist primarily of fresh fruits, leafy green vegetables, non-starchy vegetables, nuts, seeds, and whole grains. These foods are believed to be easier to digest and assimilate, thus reducing the burden on the body's detoxification systems.

Benefits of the Mucus Cleanse Diet

Proponents of the Mucus Cleanse Diet claim that adhering to its principles can lead to a wide range of health benefits. These may include improved digestion, increased energy levels, clearer skin, weight loss, reduced inflammation, and enhanced immune function. By eliminating mucus-forming foods and adopting a plant-based diet rich in nutrients and antioxidants, individuals may experience a renewed sense of vitality and well-being.

Furthermore, supporters of the Mucus Cleanse Diet argue that reducing mucus production in the body can alleviate or prevent various health conditions, including allergies, asthma, sinus congestion, bronchitis, arthritis, and digestive disorders. While scientific evidence directly supporting these claims is limited, some studies suggest that certain dietary patterns, such as plant-based diets, may indeed confer health benefits related to inflammation, oxidative stress, and chronic disease risk.

Challenges and Considerations

While the Mucus Cleanse Diet has its proponents, it also faces criticism and skepticism from mainstream health professionals and experts. Critics argue that the concept of mucus formation as the underlying cause of disease lacks scientific basis and oversimplifies complex health issues. Additionally, restricting or eliminating entire food groups, such as animal products and grains, may pose nutritional challenges and increase the risk of nutrient deficiencies if not carefully planned.

Furthermore, some individuals may find it difficult to adhere to the strict guidelines of the Mucus Cleanse Diet, especially if it requires significant changes to their usual eating habits and preferences. Social and cultural factors may also present barriers to adopting and maintaining such a dietary regimen, particularly in societies where meat and dairy consumption is deeply ingrained in culinary traditions.

Conclusion

In conclusion, the Mucus Cleanse Diet represents a holistic approach to health and wellness that emphasizes the importance of dietary choices in promoting detoxification and healing. While its principles are rooted in historical naturopathic traditions, the diet continues to attract interest from individuals seeking natural remedies for various health concerns. However, it's essential to approach any dietary regimen with caution and skepticism, taking into account individual needs, preferences, and nutritional requirements. Further research is needed to fully understand the potential benefits and limitations of the Mucus Cleanse Diet in the context of modern health science.

CHAPTER TWO

Understanding Mucus: Its Functions and Impact on Health

Mucus is a viscous, gel-like substance produced by mucous membranes throughout the body. While often associated with nasal congestion and respiratory ailments, mucus serves several important functions beyond simply trapping pathogens. Understanding its role in the body is crucial for appreciating its impact on health and its implications for various bodily systems.

Functions of Mucus

Mucus plays diverse roles in maintaining the health and function of different tissues and organs. Its primary functions include:

1. **Protection:** Mucus serves as a protective barrier, coating the surfaces of tissues to prevent them from drying out and shielding them from harmful substances, such as pathogens, pollutants, and irritants.

2. **Lubrication:** Mucus lubricates surfaces within the body, facilitating smooth movement and reducing friction between tissues and organs. For example, mucus in the gastrointestinal tract helps food move through the digestive system.

3. **Moistening:** Mucus helps maintain optimal moisture levels in various body cavities, such as the nasal passages, throat, and

respiratory tract. Adequate moisture is essential for proper function and comfort.

4. **Immune Defense:** Mucus contains immune cells, antibodies, and antimicrobial compounds that help defend against infections by trapping and neutralizing pathogens, such as bacteria, viruses, and fungi.

5. **Clearance:** Mucus aids in the removal of foreign particles, debris, and microorganisms from the body by trapping them and facilitating their expulsion through coughing, sneezing, swallowing, or expectoration.

Impact of Mucus on Health

While mucus serves vital functions in the body, abnormalities in its production, composition, or clearance can have significant implications for health. Excessive or thickened mucus, for example, can lead to congestion, discomfort, and respiratory symptoms. Conversely, inadequate mucus production or impaired clearance can increase the risk of infections and compromise tissue integrity.

Respiratory Health: In the respiratory system, mucus plays a critical role in defending against airborne pathogens and irritants. Conditions such as colds, flu, allergies, and respiratory infections can cause mucus overproduction and congestion, leading to symptoms such as nasal congestion, coughing, and throat irritation. Chronic respiratory conditions like asthma, chronic obstructive pulmonary disease (COPD), and cystic fibrosis can also affect mucus production and clearance, contributing to recurrent infections and breathing difficulties.

Digestive Health: Mucus production in the gastrointestinal tract is essential for lubricating the digestive lining, protecting against stomach acid, and aiding in the passage of food. However, disruptions in mucus production or composition can contribute to digestive disorders such as gastritis, gastroesophageal reflux disease (GERD), inflammatory bowel disease (IBD), and ulcers. In these conditions, alterations in mucus quality or quantity may compromise the protective barrier of the digestive tract, leading to inflammation, ulceration, and impaired nutrient absorption.

Reproductive Health: Mucus also plays a role in reproductive health, particularly in the female reproductive system. Cervical mucus undergoes cyclic changes in response to hormonal fluctuations throughout the menstrual cycle, affecting fertility and facilitating sperm transport. Abnormalities in cervical mucus production or consistency can interfere with conception and fertility.

Skin Health: Mucus secretion by glands in the skin helps maintain hydration, protect against pathogens, and facilitate wound healing. However, excessive mucus production or altered skin mucus composition can contribute to skin conditions such as acne, eczema, and psoriasis.

Conclusion

In conclusion, mucus is a multifunctional substance with diverse roles in maintaining the health and function of various tissues and organs throughout the body. Its functions extend beyond mere lubrication and include protection, immune defense, and clearance of foreign particles. Abnormalities in mucus production, composition, or clearance can have significant implications for respiratory, digestive, reproductive, and skin health, contributing to a range of disorders and symptoms. Understanding the complex interplay between mucus and health is essential for developing effective strategies for prevention, diagnosis, and treatment of mucus-related conditions.

CHAPTER THREE

The Role of Herbal Remedies in Detoxification

Detoxification, the process of eliminating toxins and waste products from the body, has been a fundamental concept in traditional medicine systems for centuries. While the body has its own natural detoxification mechanisms, proponents of detox diets and cleansing regimens often turn to herbal remedies to support and enhance these processes. Herbal remedies, derived from plants and botanicals, are believed to offer a range of detoxifying benefits, including aiding liver function, promoting digestion, and supporting the elimination of toxins through various organs of elimination.

Historical Context

Herbal remedies have been used for detoxification purposes in traditional medicine systems such as Ayurveda, Traditional Chinese Medicine (TCM), and Indigenous healing practices for thousands of years. These systems recognize the importance of supporting the body's natural detoxification processes to maintain health and vitality. Herbs and botanicals have been prized for their ability to stimulate organ function, purify the blood, and promote the elimination of waste products accumulated in the body.

Herbal Remedies for Detoxification

Numerous herbs and botanicals are believed to possess detoxifying properties and have been traditionally used for this purpose. Some of the most commonly utilized herbs in detoxification protocols include:

1. **Dandelion (Taraxacum officinale):** Dandelion is prized for its diuretic properties, which may help flush toxins from the kidneys and promote urine production. It is also believed to support liver function and stimulate bile production, aiding in the digestion and elimination of fats and toxins.

2. **Milk Thistle (Silybum marianum):** Milk thistle contains compounds known as silymarin, which have potent antioxidant and hepatoprotective properties. It is commonly used to support liver health and protect against damage from toxins, pollutants, and alcohol.

3. **Burdock Root (Arctium lappa):** Burdock root is revered for its blood-purifying properties and is traditionally used to eliminate toxins from the blood and lymphatic system. It is also believed to support liver and kidney function, aiding in detoxification.

4. **Ginger (Zingiber officinale):** Ginger is valued for its digestive properties, helping to alleviate nausea, bloating, and indigestion. It may also stimulate circulation and promote

sweating, facilitating the elimination of toxins through the skin.

5. **Turmeric (Curcuma longa):** Turmeric contains the active compound curcumin, which exhibits potent anti-inflammatory and antioxidant properties. It is believed to support liver function, enhance bile production, and aid in detoxification processes.

6. **Nettle (Urtica dioica):** Nettle is rich in vitamins, minerals, and antioxidants, making it a popular choice for detoxification protocols. It is traditionally used to support kidney function, promote urine production, and remove waste products from the body.

7. **Licorice Root (Glycyrrhiza glabra):** Licorice root is valued for its soothing properties and is traditionally used to support adrenal health and enhance detoxification processes. It may also help alleviate symptoms of gastrointestinal distress and promote liver function.

Mechanisms of Action

Herbal remedies exert their detoxifying effects through various mechanisms, including:

- **Liver Support:** Many herbs support liver function by enhancing detoxification pathways, promoting bile production, and protecting liver cells from damage.

- **Kidney Support:** Certain herbs have diuretic properties, increasing urine production and facilitating the elimination of toxins through the kidneys.

- **Antioxidant Activity:** Herbs rich in antioxidants help neutralize free radicals and reduce oxidative stress, protecting cells and tissues from damage caused by toxins and pollutants.

- **Anti-inflammatory Effects:** Some herbs have anti-inflammatory properties, reducing inflammation and supporting the body's natural detoxification processes.

- **Digestive Support:** Many herbs aid digestion by promoting the production of digestive enzymes, stimulating bile flow, and relieving gastrointestinal symptoms such as bloating and indigestion.

Considerations and Precautions

While herbal remedies can offer valuable support for detoxification, it's essential to use them judiciously and under the guidance of a qualified healthcare practitioner, particularly if you have underlying health conditions or are taking medications. Some herbs may interact with medications or exacerbate certain health issues, so it's important to seek personalized advice before incorporating them into your regimen.

Additionally, herbal remedies should be used as part of a comprehensive approach to detoxification, which includes adopting a healthy diet, staying hydrated, engaging in regular physical activity, and minimizing exposure to environmental toxins. Detoxification should be approached with caution, as extreme or prolonged detox regimens may disrupt the body's natural balance and lead to adverse effects.

In conclusion, herbal remedies play a valuable role in supporting detoxification processes by promoting liver and kidney function, enhancing digestion, and reducing oxidative stress. When used appropriately and as part of a holistic approach to wellness, herbs can contribute to overall health and vitality. However, it's essential to consult with a healthcare professional to determine the most appropriate herbs and dosages for your individual needs and circumstances.

CHAPTER FOUR

Preparing Your Body for the Cleanse: Pre-Cleanse Phase

Embarking on a cleanse or detoxification program can be an effective way to reset your body, eliminate toxins, and promote overall health and well-being. However, to maximize the benefits of the cleanse and minimize potential side effects, it's essential to prepare your body adequately beforehand. The pre-cleanse phase is a crucial step in this process, focusing on gradually transitioning to a cleaner diet, hydrating the body, and mentally preparing for the upcoming cleanse.

Assessing Your Readiness

Before starting any cleanse or detox program, it's important to assess your readiness and suitability for the process. Consider factors such as your current diet, lifestyle habits, medical history, and any underlying health conditions. If you have any concerns or medical issues, consult with a healthcare professional before beginning the cleanse to ensure it is safe and appropriate for you.

Gradual Transition to Clean Eating

Transitioning to a cleaner diet in the days or weeks leading up to the cleanse can help prepare your body for the process and reduce the likelihood of experiencing detox symptoms. Focus on gradually eliminating processed foods, refined sugars, caffeine, alcohol, and other dietary toxins from your diet. Instead, emphasize whole, nutrient-dense foods such as fruits, vegetables, whole grains, legumes, nuts, seeds, and lean proteins.

Hydration

Proper hydration is essential for supporting the body's natural detoxification processes and optimizing overall health. Increase your water intake in the days leading up to the cleanse to ensure adequate hydration. Aim to drink at least eight glasses of water per day, and consider incorporating hydrating foods such as water-rich fruits and vegetables into your diet.

Supporting Liver Function

The liver plays a central role in detoxification, metabolizing and eliminating toxins from the body. Supporting liver function during the pre-cleanse phase can help enhance the effectiveness of the cleanse. Incorporate liver-supportive foods and herbs into your diet, such as cruciferous vegetables (e.g., broccoli, Brussels sprouts, kale), garlic, onions, turmeric, dandelion root, milk thistle, and burdock root.

Elimination of Trigger Foods

Identify and eliminate potential trigger foods or allergens from your diet during the pre-cleanse phase. Common trigger foods include gluten, dairy, soy, corn, eggs, and nuts. By avoiding these foods, you can reduce inflammation, support digestion, and minimize potential adverse reactions during the cleanse.

Mindful Eating and Stress Management

Practicing mindful eating and stress management techniques during the pre-cleanse phase can help prepare your body and mind for the cleanse. Slow down during meals, chew your food thoroughly, and savor each bite. Minimize distractions and cultivate a sense of gratitude for the nourishment you are providing your body. Additionally, engage in stress-reducing activities such as yoga, meditation, deep breathing exercises, or spending time in nature to promote relaxation and emotional well-being.

Setting Intentions

Set clear intentions for the cleanse and visualize the outcomes you hope to achieve. Whether your goals are physical, mental, or emotional, clarifying your intentions can provide motivation and focus throughout the process. Write down your intentions in a journal or create a vision board to reinforce your commitment to the cleanse.

Conclusion

The pre-cleanse phase is a vital component of any detoxification program, laying the foundation for a successful and effective cleanse. By gradually transitioning to a cleaner diet, hydrating the body, supporting liver function, eliminating trigger foods, practicing mindful eating, and setting intentions, you can prepare your body and mind for the cleansing process ahead. Approach the pre-cleanse phase with patience, self-care, and a positive mindset, knowing that you are taking proactive steps toward improving your health and well-being.

CHAPTER FIVE

Dr. Barbara's Herbal Mucus Cleanse Diet Plan: Step-by-Step Guide

Dr. Barbara's Herbal Mucus Cleanse Diet Plan offers a holistic approach to detoxification and improving overall health by targeting the reduction of mucus-forming foods and incorporating herbal remedies known for their detoxifying properties. This step-by-step guide outlines the key principles and strategies for implementing Dr. Barbara's cleanse effectively.

Step 1: Pre-Cleanse Preparation

Before beginning the cleanse, take time to prepare your body and mind for the process. Gradually transition to a cleaner diet by eliminating processed foods, refined sugars, caffeine, alcohol, and other dietary toxins. Focus on consuming whole, nutrient-dense foods such as fruits, vegetables, whole grains, legumes, nuts, seeds, and lean proteins. Increase your water intake to ensure proper hydration, and incorporate liver-supportive foods and herbs into your diet, such as cruciferous vegetables, garlic, turmeric, dandelion root, and milk thistle.

Step 2: Herbal Protocol Selection

Consult with Dr. Barbara or a qualified herbalist to determine the most appropriate herbal protocol for your individual needs and health goals. Dr. Barbara's Herbal Mucus Cleanse may include a combination of herbs and botanicals known for their detoxifying and mucus-reducing properties. Common herbs used in the cleanse may include dandelion root, milk thistle, burdock root, ginger, turmeric, nettle, and licorice root. These herbs may be consumed in various forms, including teas, tinctures, capsules, or powdered supplements.

Step 3: Elimination of Mucus-Forming Foods

During the cleanse, focus on eliminating mucus-forming foods from your diet to reduce mucus production and support detoxification. These may include animal products such as meat, dairy, and eggs, as well as refined grains, processed foods, and certain fruits and vegetables high in starch or sugar. Instead, emphasize mucusless foods such as fresh fruits, leafy green vegetables, non-starchy vegetables, nuts, seeds, and whole grains. Be mindful of food sensitivities or allergies and avoid trigger foods that may exacerbate mucus production or inflammation.

Step 4: Herbal Supplementation and Detox Protocols

Follow the prescribed herbal supplementation and detox protocols as recommended by Dr. Barbara or your healthcare provider. This may involve consuming herbal teas, tinctures, or supplements at specified times throughout the day to support liver function, promote digestion, and enhance the elimination of toxins. Be consistent with your herbal regimen and adhere to the recommended dosage guidelines to maximize the benefits of the cleanse.

Step 5: Hydration and Fluid Intake

Stay hydrated throughout the cleanse by drinking plenty of water and herbal teas to support the body's natural detoxification processes. Aim to drink at least eight glasses of water per day, and consider incorporating hydrating foods such as water-rich fruits and vegetables into your diet. Proper hydration is essential for flushing toxins from the body and maintaining optimal health and well-being.

Step 6: Mindful Eating and Self-Care Practices

Practice mindful eating and self-care practices to support your physical, mental, and emotional well-being during the cleanse. Slow down during meals, chew your food thoroughly, and savor each bite. Prioritize relaxation and stress management techniques such as yoga, meditation, deep breathing exercises, or spending time in nature to promote relaxation and emotional balance. Listen to your body's cues and honor its needs throughout the cleansing process.

Step 7: Post-Cleanse Integration and Maintenance

After completing the cleanse, gradually reintroduce foods into your diet while paying attention to how your body responds. Take note of any symptoms or reactions and make adjustments as needed to maintain a balanced and healthful eating pattern. Continue to incorporate liver-supportive foods and herbs into your diet, and practice mindful eating and self-care practices to support long-term health and well-being. Consider periodic cleanses or detox protocols as part of your ongoing health maintenance routine.

Conclusion

Dr. Barbara's Herbal Mucus Cleanse Diet Plan offers a comprehensive approach to detoxification and improving overall health by targeting mucus reduction and supporting the body's natural detoxification processes. By following this step-by-step guide and incorporating herbal remedies, dietary modifications, hydration, mindful eating, and self-care practices, you can promote detoxification, enhance vitality, and achieve optimal health and well-being. Consult with Dr. Barbara or a qualified healthcare provider before beginning any cleanse or detox program to ensure it is safe and appropriate for your individual needs and health status.

CHAPTER SIX

The Power of Herbs: Key Ingredients in the Cleanse

Herbs have long been recognized for their potent medicinal properties and their ability to support the body's natural detoxification processes. In Dr. Barbara's Herbal Mucus Cleanse Diet Plan, several key ingredients are incorporated for their detoxifying, anti-inflammatory, and mucus-reducing properties. These herbs play a crucial role in promoting overall health and well-being during the cleanse. Let's explore some of the key ingredients and their therapeutic benefits:

1. Dandelion Root (Taraxacum officinale):

- **Liver Support:** Dandelion root is prized for its ability to support liver function, enhance bile production, and promote detoxification. It contains bitter compounds known as taraxacin and taraxacerin, which stimulate bile flow and aid in the elimination of toxins from the liver.

- **Diuretic Properties:** Dandelion root acts as a natural diuretic, increasing urine production and promoting the elimination of waste products and excess fluids from the body. This helps reduce bloating, water retention, and swelling.

2. Milk Thistle (Silybum marianum):

- **Hepatoprotective Effects:** Milk thistle contains a flavonoid complex called silymarin, which has potent antioxidant and anti-inflammatory properties. It helps protect liver cells from damage caused by toxins, pollutants, and free radicals, thereby supporting liver health and function.

- **Detoxification Support:** Silymarin enhances the liver's ability to detoxify harmful substances by increasing the production of glutathione, a powerful antioxidant that aids in the neutralization and elimination of toxins.

3. Burdock Root (Arctium lappa):

- **Blood Purification:** Burdock root is renowned for its blood-purifying properties, helping to eliminate toxins and waste products from the bloodstream. It contains compounds called lignans, which have been shown to support detoxification and enhance the elimination of metabolic waste.

- **Lymphatic Support:** Burdock root supports lymphatic drainage and circulation, aiding in the removal of cellular waste and toxins from the body's tissues. It helps reduce congestion and inflammation in the lymphatic system, promoting overall detoxification and immune function.

4. Ginger (Zingiber officinale):

- **Digestive Support:** Ginger is valued for its digestive properties, helping to alleviate nausea, bloating, indigestion, and gastrointestinal discomfort. It stimulates digestion, promotes gastric motility, and enhances nutrient absorption.

- **Anti-inflammatory Effects:** Ginger contains bioactive compounds such as gingerol and shogaol, which exhibit potent anti-inflammatory and antioxidant properties. It helps reduce inflammation in the digestive tract and throughout the body, supporting overall health and well-being.

5. Turmeric (Curcuma longa):

- **Anti-inflammatory Activity:** Turmeric contains curcumin, a bioactive compound with powerful anti-inflammatory and antioxidant properties. It helps reduce inflammation, oxidative stress, and tissue damage caused by toxins and free radicals.

- **Liver Protection:** Curcumin supports liver health by enhancing antioxidant defenses, promoting bile production, and reducing inflammation in the liver. It helps protect against liver damage and supports detoxification processes.

6. Nettle (Urtica dioica):

- **Nutrient-Rich:** Nettle is rich in vitamins, minerals, and antioxidants, making it a valuable addition to the cleanse. It provides essential nutrients that support overall health and vitality during the detoxification process.

- **Diuretic Properties:** Nettle acts as a gentle diuretic, promoting urine production and facilitating the elimination of toxins from the body. It helps reduce fluid retention, bloating, and swelling, supporting kidney function and detoxification.

Conclusion

The key ingredients in Dr. Barbara's Herbal Mucus Cleanse Diet Plan offer a powerful combination of detoxifying, anti-inflammatory, and health-promoting properties. By incorporating these herbs into the cleanse, you can support liver function, promote digestion, reduce inflammation, and enhance overall detoxification and well-being. Consult with Dr. Barbara or a qualified healthcare provider to determine the most appropriate herbal protocol for your individual needs and health goals.

CHAPTER SEVEN

Managing Detox Symptoms and Side Effects Safely

Embarking on a cleanse or detoxification program can sometimes lead to temporary side effects and detox symptoms as the body adjusts to dietary changes and eliminates toxins. While these symptoms are often a natural part of the cleansing process, it's essential to manage them safely and effectively to minimize discomfort and support overall well-being. Here are some strategies for managing detox symptoms and side effects safely:

1. Stay Hydrated: Proper hydration is essential for supporting the body's natural detoxification processes and minimizing detox symptoms. Drink plenty of water throughout the day to flush toxins from the body and maintain optimal hydration levels. Herbal teas, coconut water, and electrolyte-rich beverages can also help replenish fluids and support detoxification.

2. Eat Nutrient-Dense Foods: Focus on consuming nutrient-dense foods that support detoxification and provide essential vitamins, minerals, and antioxidants. Incorporate plenty of fruits, vegetables, whole grains, legumes, nuts, seeds, and lean proteins into your diet to nourish your body and support overall health. Avoid processed foods, refined sugars, and artificial additives that may exacerbate detox symptoms.

3. Support Liver Health: The liver plays a central role in detoxification, metabolizing and eliminating toxins from the body. Support liver function by consuming liver-supportive foods and herbs such as dandelion root, milk thistle, turmeric, and burdock root. These herbs help enhance bile production, promote liver detoxification pathways, and protect liver cells from damage caused by toxins and free radicals.

4. Practice Gentle Exercise: Engage in gentle exercise such as walking, yoga, tai chi, or swimming to promote circulation, lymphatic drainage, and the elimination of toxins through sweat. Exercise also helps reduce stress, support digestion, and improve overall well-being. Listen to your body and choose activities that feel comfortable and energizing during the cleanse.

5. Get Plenty of Rest: Adequate rest and relaxation are essential for supporting the body's detoxification processes and minimizing detox symptoms. Aim for seven to nine hours of quality sleep each night to allow your body to repair, regenerate, and detoxify. Practice relaxation techniques such as meditation, deep breathing exercises, or gentle stretching before bedtime to promote restful sleep and reduce stress.

6. Manage Stress: Chronic stress can impair detoxification pathways and exacerbate detox symptoms. Take time to manage stress effectively by practicing stress-reducing techniques such as meditation, mindfulness, progressive muscle relaxation, or spending time in nature. Prioritize self-care activities that promote relaxation, balance, and emotional well-being during the cleanse.

7. Listen to Your Body: Pay attention to your body's signals and adjust your cleanse protocol as needed to minimize discomfort and support overall well-being. If you experience severe or prolonged detox symptoms, consider slowing down the cleanse, incorporating more nourishing foods, or consulting with a healthcare professional for personalized guidance and support.

8. Gradual Transition: After completing the cleanse, gradually reintroduce foods into your diet while paying attention to how your body responds. Take note of any symptoms or reactions and make adjustments as needed to maintain a balanced and healthful eating pattern. Focus on incorporating whole, nutrient-dense foods that support long-term health and well-being.

Conclusion

Managing detox symptoms and side effects safely is an essential aspect of any cleanse or detoxification program. By staying hydrated, eating nutrient-dense foods, supporting liver health, practicing gentle exercise, getting plenty of rest, managing stress, listening to your body, and gradually transitioning after the cleanse, you can minimize discomfort and support overall well-being during the detoxification process. Remember to consult with a healthcare professional before beginning any cleanse or detox program, especially if you have underlying health conditions or concerns.

CHAPTER EIGHT

Incorporating Exercise and Stress Management into Your Cleanse

Exercise and stress management play crucial roles in supporting overall health and well-being, especially during a cleanse or detoxification program. Incorporating regular physical activity and stress-reducing practices can enhance the effectiveness of the cleanse, support detoxification processes, and promote holistic wellness. Here's how to integrate exercise and stress management into your cleanse:

1. Choose Gentle Exercise: During a cleanse, focus on gentle forms of exercise that promote circulation, lymphatic drainage, and detoxification without placing undue stress on the body. Options include walking, yoga, tai chi, qigong, swimming, and cycling. These activities help stimulate the body's natural detoxification processes, support digestion, and improve overall well-being.

2. Establish a Routine: Set aside dedicated time for exercise each day, incorporating it into your cleanse schedule. Aim for at least 30 minutes of moderate-intensity exercise most days of the week, gradually increasing duration and intensity as tolerated. Consistency is key to reaping the benefits of exercise during the cleanse.

3. Practice Mindful Movement: Pay attention to your body's signals and practice mindful movement during exercise. Focus on proper form, alignment, and breathing to enhance relaxation, reduce stress, and promote body awareness. Mind-body practices such as yoga and tai chi emphasize mindfulness, breathwork, and gentle movement, making them ideal for incorporating into your cleanse routine.

4. Engage in Outdoor Activities: Take advantage of the healing power of nature by exercising outdoors whenever possible. Spending time in nature has been shown to reduce stress, improve mood, and enhance overall well-being. Choose activities such as hiking, jogging, or walking in natural settings to reap the benefits of outdoor exercise during the cleanse.

5. Prioritize Stress Reduction: Chronic stress can impair detoxification processes and undermine the effectiveness of the cleanse. Incorporate stress-reducing practices into your daily routine to promote relaxation, emotional balance, and overall well-being. Options include meditation, deep breathing exercises, progressive muscle relaxation, guided imagery, and mindfulness practices.

6. Schedule Regular Breaks: Take regular breaks throughout the day to rest, recharge, and engage in stress-reducing activities. Set aside time for relaxation practices such as meditation, deep breathing, or gentle stretching to help alleviate tension, reduce stress hormones, and promote a sense of calm during the cleanse.

7. Create a Supportive Environment: Surround yourself with supportive people and environments that promote relaxation, positivity, and well-being. Seek out social connections, join support groups, or participate in wellness activities that align with your cleanse goals. Having a strong support network can provide encouragement, motivation, and accountability throughout the cleansing process.

8. Listen to Your Body: Pay attention to your body's cues and adjust your exercise and stress management practices as needed to support your overall well-being during the cleanse. If you experience fatigue, discomfort, or other signs of overexertion, scale back your exercise intensity or duration, and prioritize rest and recovery.

9. Stay Hydrated: Drink plenty of water before, during, and after exercise to stay hydrated and support the body's detoxification processes. Proper hydration is essential for maintaining energy levels, regulating body temperature, and flushing toxins from the body.

10. Practice Self-Care: Incorporate self-care practices into your daily routine to nurture your body, mind, and spirit during the cleanse. Prioritize activities that promote relaxation, pleasure, and enjoyment, such as taking a warm bath, indulging in a massage, reading a book, or spending time in nature.

Conclusion

Integrating exercise and stress management practices into your cleanse can enhance detoxification, support overall health and well-being, and promote a sense of balance and vitality. By choosing gentle forms of exercise, establishing a routine, practicing mindful movement, engaging in outdoor activities, prioritizing stress reduction, scheduling regular breaks, creating a supportive environment, listening to your body, staying hydrated, and practicing self-care, you can optimize the effectiveness of your cleanse and cultivate a healthier, more vibrant lifestyle. Remember to consult with a healthcare professional before beginning any new exercise or stress management regimen, especially if you have underlying health conditions or concerns.

CHAPTER NINE

Transitioning Out of the Cleanse: Post-Cleanse Guidelines

Completing a cleanse or detoxification program is an accomplishment, but transitioning back to a regular diet and lifestyle is equally important for maintaining the benefits of the cleanse and promoting long-term health and well-being. The post-cleanse phase is a critical period during which you reintroduce foods gradually, support digestion, and continue to prioritize healthy habits. Here are some guidelines for transitioning out of the cleanse effectively:

1. Gradual Food Reintroduction:

- Begin by reintroducing foods gradually, starting with easily digestible options such as steamed vegetables, soups, and salads.

- Monitor your body's response to each food reintroduction, paying attention to any signs of digestive discomfort, bloating, or adverse reactions.

- Slowly reintroduce potential trigger foods such as gluten, dairy, soy, and processed foods, and observe how your body reacts. Consider keeping a food diary to track your responses.

2. Emphasize Whole, Nutrient-Dense Foods:

- Focus on incorporating whole, nutrient-dense foods into your diet, including fruits, vegetables, whole grains, legumes, nuts, seeds, and lean proteins.

- Choose organic, locally sourced, and minimally processed foods whenever possible to maximize nutritional quality and minimize exposure to pesticides and additives.

3. Support Digestive Health:

- Continue to support digestive health by consuming fiber-rich foods, fermented foods, and prebiotic-rich foods that nourish beneficial gut bacteria.

- Incorporate digestive aids such as probiotics, digestive enzymes, and herbal teas to support digestion, reduce bloating, and enhance nutrient absorption.

4. Hydrate Adequately:

- Maintain proper hydration by drinking plenty of water throughout the day. Aim to consume at least eight glasses of water daily to support detoxification, digestion, and overall health.

- Incorporate hydrating foods such as water-rich fruits and vegetables, herbal teas, and coconut water to replenish fluids and electrolytes.

5. Continue Liver Support:

- Support liver health and detoxification processes by incorporating liver-supportive foods and herbs into your diet. Include foods such as cruciferous vegetables, garlic, onions, turmeric, dandelion root, and milk thistle.

- Limit exposure to environmental toxins and pollutants by choosing organic produce, using natural cleaning and personal care products, and minimizing exposure to air and water contaminants.

6. Maintain Healthy Habits:

- Continue to prioritize healthy habits such as regular exercise, stress management, adequate sleep, and self-care practices to support overall health and well-being.

- Engage in regular physical activity, including aerobic exercise, strength training, flexibility exercises, and mind-body practices such as yoga, tai chi, or meditation.

7. Listen to Your Body:

- Pay attention to your body's signals and adjust your diet and lifestyle as needed to support your overall well-being. If you experience digestive discomfort, fatigue, or other symptoms, consider revisiting your dietary choices and lifestyle habits.

8. Reflect on Your Experience:

- Take time to reflect on your cleanse experience and the lessons learned. Consider what aspects of the cleanse were most beneficial for you and how you can incorporate them into your ongoing health routine.

- Celebrate your accomplishments and acknowledge the progress you've made toward improving your health and well-being through the cleanse process.

9. Set Intentions for Continued Health:

- Set intentions for maintaining your health and well-being beyond the cleanse. Establish realistic goals and action steps for incorporating healthy habits into your daily life and making sustainable lifestyle changes.

- Stay connected to your motivation and commitment to health by regularly revisiting your goals and intentions, and making adjustments as needed to stay on track.

10. Seek Support if Needed:

- If you encounter challenges or need additional guidance during the post-cleanse phase, don't hesitate to seek support from a healthcare professional, nutritionist, or wellness coach. They can provide personalized recommendations and assistance to help you navigate this transition period successfully.

Conclusion: Transitioning out of the cleanse is a crucial phase in the detoxification process, during which you reintroduce foods gradually, support digestion, and continue to prioritize healthy habits. By following these post-cleanse guidelines and listening to your body's signals, you can maintain the benefits of the cleanse and cultivate a healthier, more vibrant lifestyle over the long term. Remember that the journey to optimal health is ongoing, and each step you take toward wellness is a valuable investment in your well-being.

CHAPTER TEN

Long-Term Benefits and Maintenance Strategies for Optimal Health

Embarking on a cleanse or detoxification program can offer immediate benefits such as improved energy, mental clarity, and digestive function. However, the true value lies in sustaining these benefits over the long term and cultivating a lifestyle that supports optimal health and well-being. Here are some long-term benefits of cleansing and maintenance strategies for achieving and maintaining optimal health:

1. Enhanced Detoxification and Cleansing:

- Regular cleansing supports the body's natural detoxification processes, helping to eliminate accumulated toxins, pollutants, and metabolic waste products. By incorporating periodic cleanses into your wellness routine, you can optimize detoxification pathways and promote overall health and vitality.

2. Improved Digestive Health:

- Cleansing programs often emphasize digestive support and elimination of foods that may contribute to digestive discomfort and inflammation. By adopting a diet rich in fiber, probiotics, and digestive enzymes, you can maintain optimal digestive function, support gut health, and reduce the risk of digestive issues such as bloating, gas, and constipation.

3. Enhanced Nutrient Absorption:

- Cleansing programs promote the consumption of nutrient-dense foods that provide essential vitamins, minerals, antioxidants, and phytonutrients. By supporting optimal digestion and absorption of nutrients, you can ensure that your body receives the essential building blocks it needs for cellular repair, immune function, and overall health.

4. Weight Management:

- Cleansing programs often result in temporary weight loss due to the elimination of processed foods, refined sugars, and excess calories. By adopting a balanced and healthful diet and incorporating regular physical activity into your routine, you can achieve and maintain a healthy weight over the long term.

5. Enhanced Energy and Vitality:

- Cleansing programs help reset the body's energy systems, leading to improved energy levels, mental clarity, and overall vitality. By prioritizing rest, hydration, nutrient-rich foods, and stress management techniques, you can sustain high energy levels and support optimal physical and mental performance.

6. Reduced Inflammation and Oxidative Stress:

- Cleansing programs often emphasize anti-inflammatory and antioxidant-rich foods and herbs that help reduce inflammation and oxidative stress in the body. By minimizing exposure to inflammatory foods and environmental toxins and maximizing intake of antioxidant-rich foods, you can support cellular health and reduce the risk of chronic diseases associated with inflammation and oxidative damage.

7. Strengthened Immune Function:

- Cleansing programs support immune function by promoting the elimination of toxins and pathogens from the body and enhancing the body's natural defenses. By adopting a nutrient-rich diet, managing stress, getting adequate sleep, and engaging in regular physical activity, you can support immune health and reduce the risk of infections and illness.

Maintenance Strategies for Optimal Health:

1. Balanced and Nutrient-Rich Diet:

- Emphasize whole, nutrient-dense foods such as fruits, vegetables, whole grains, legumes, nuts, seeds, and lean proteins. Aim to consume a variety of colors, textures, and flavors to ensure a wide range of nutrients and phytonutrients.

2. Regular Physical Activity:

- Engage in regular exercise, including aerobic activity, strength training, flexibility exercises, and mind-body practices such as yoga or tai chi. Aim for at least 150 minutes of moderate-intensity exercise or 75 minutes of vigorous-intensity exercise per week, as recommended by health guidelines.

3. Stress Management:

- Prioritize stress-reducing practices such as meditation, deep breathing exercises, progressive muscle relaxation, or spending time in nature. Incorporate relaxation techniques into your daily routine to promote emotional balance, reduce stress hormones, and support overall well-being.

4. Hydration:

- Stay hydrated by drinking plenty of water throughout the day. Aim to consume at least eight glasses of water daily, and incorporate hydrating foods such as water-rich fruits and vegetables, herbal teas, and coconut water.

5. Quality Sleep:

- Prioritize quality sleep by establishing a consistent sleep schedule, creating a relaxing bedtime routine, and optimizing your sleep environment. Aim for seven to nine hours of sleep per night to support cellular repair, cognitive function, and overall health.

6. Mindful Eating:

- Practice mindful eating by paying attention to hunger and satiety cues, chewing food thoroughly, and savoring each bite. Eat slowly, without distractions, and cultivate a sense of gratitude for the nourishment you are providing your body.

7. Regular Health Check-Ups:

- Schedule regular health check-ups with your healthcare provider to monitor key health markers such as blood pressure, cholesterol levels, blood sugar levels, and body weight. Discuss any concerns or symptoms with your healthcare provider and follow their recommendations for preventive care and screenings.

8. Continuous Learning and Self-Reflection:

- Stay informed about the latest research and developments in nutrition, exercise, and wellness by reading books, attending seminars, and following reputable sources of health information. Engage in self-reflection and continuous learning to deepen your understanding of your body's needs and preferences.

Conclusion: Achieving and maintaining optimal health requires a holistic approach that encompasses nutrition, exercise, stress management, sleep, hydration, and self-care practices. By incorporating long-term maintenance strategies into your daily routine and staying committed to your health goals, you can cultivate a vibrant and fulfilling life and enjoy the benefits of optimal health for years to come. Remember that small, consistent changes over time can lead to significant improvements in your health and well-being.

CHAPTER 11

RECIPES FOR MUCUS CLEANSE

1. Peppermint Tea

- **Definition:** Peppermint tea is a herbal infusion made from peppermint leaves, known for its soothing properties.

- **Ingredients:** Fresh peppermint leaves or dried peppermint, hot water.

- **How to Prepare:** Steep peppermint leaves in hot water for 5-10 minutes.

- **How to Use:** Drink 1-2 cups daily.

- **Dosage:** 1-2 cups per day.

- **Side Effects:** Peppermint tea is generally safe but may cause heartburn in some individuals.

- **Precautions:** Avoid if you have gastroesophageal reflux disease (GERD) or hiatal hernia.

2. Ginger-Lemon-Honey Tea

- **Definition:** A warming tea blend that helps soothe the throat and clear mucus.

- **Ingredients:** Fresh ginger, lemon juice, honey, hot water.

- **How to Prepare:** Grate ginger, add lemon juice, honey, and hot water.

- **How to Use:** Drink 1-2 cups daily.

- **Dosage:** 1-2 cups per day.

- **Side Effects:** May cause heartburn or digestive discomfort in some individuals.

- **Precautions:** Avoid excessive consumption if you have gallstone disease.

3. Turmeric Milk

- **Definition:** A traditional Ayurvedic remedy known for its anti-inflammatory properties.

- **Ingredients:** Turmeric powder, milk, honey.

- **How to Prepare:** Heat milk, add turmeric powder and honey.

- **How to Use:** Drink before bedtime.

- **Dosage:** 1 cup before bedtime.

- **Side Effects:** Rarely, may cause allergic reactions or digestive issues.

- **Precautions:** Avoid if you have bile duct obstruction or gallstones.

4. Eucalyptus Steam Inhalation

- **Definition:** Inhalation of eucalyptus steam to clear nasal passages.

- **Ingredients:** Eucalyptus leaves or oil, hot water.

- **How to Prepare:** Add eucalyptus leaves or oil to hot water, inhale steam.

- **How to Use:** Inhale steam for 5-10 minutes.

- **Dosage:** Use as needed.

- **Side Effects:** Inhalation may cause irritation in sensitive individuals.

- **Precautions:** Avoid direct contact with eyes; discontinue if irritation occurs.

5. Nettle Leaf Tea

- **Definition:** Nettle leaf tea helps reduce inflammation and supports respiratory health.

- **Ingredients:** Dried nettle leaves, hot water.

- **How to Prepare:** Steep dried nettle leaves in hot water for 5-10 minutes.

- **How to Use:** Drink 1-2 cups daily.

- **Dosage:** 1-2 cups per day.

- **Side Effects:** May cause mild stomach upset or allergic reactions.

- **Precautions:** Avoid if pregnant, breastfeeding, or taking blood thinners.

6. Licorice Root Tea

- **Definition:** Licorice root tea helps soothe throat irritation and reduce mucus production.

- **Ingredients:** Dried licorice root, hot water.

- **How to Prepare:** Steep dried licorice root in hot water for 5-10 minutes.

- **How to Use:** Drink 1-2 cups daily.

- **Dosage:** 1-2 cups per day.

- **Side Effects:** Prolonged use may lead to high blood pressure or potassium imbalance.

- **Precautions:** Avoid if you have high blood pressure or kidney disease.

7. Fenugreek Tea

- **Definition:** Fenugreek tea helps relieve congestion and reduce mucus buildup.

- **Ingredients:** Fenugreek seeds, hot water.

- **How to Prepare:** Steep fenugreek seeds in hot water for 5-10 minutes.

- **How to Use:** Drink 1-2 cups daily.

- **Dosage:** 1-2 cups per day.

- **Side Effects:** May cause allergic reactions or gastrointestinal upset in some individuals.

- **Precautions:** Avoid if pregnant, breastfeeding, or allergic to legumes.

8. Garlic and Honey Infusion

- **Definition:** A potent antibacterial and antiviral infusion to support immune health.

- **Ingredients:** Crushed garlic cloves, honey.

- **How to Prepare:** Mix crushed garlic cloves with honey.

- **How to Use:** Consume 1 teaspoon daily.

- **Dosage:** 1 teaspoon per day.

- **Side Effects:** May cause heartburn or digestive discomfort.

- **Precautions:** Avoid if allergic to garlic or honey.

9. Cayenne Pepper Lemonade

- **Definition:** A spicy lemonade to help thin mucus and promote detoxification.

- **Ingredients:** Lemon juice, cayenne pepper, water, maple syrup.

- **How to Prepare:** Mix lemon juice, cayenne pepper, water, and maple syrup.

- **How to Use:** Drink throughout the day.

- **Dosage:** As desired throughout the day.

- **Side Effects:** May cause stomach irritation or heartburn.

- **Precautions:** Avoid if you have gastrointestinal issues or are sensitive to spicy foods.

10. **Thyme Tea**

- **Definition:** Thyme tea helps soothe coughs and congestion.

- **Ingredients:** Fresh or dried thyme leaves, hot water.

- **How to Prepare:** Steep thyme leaves in hot water for 5-10 minutes.

- **How to Use:** Drink 1-2 cups daily.

- **Dosage:** 1-2 cups per day.

- **Side Effects:** Rarely, may cause allergic reactions or digestive upset.

- **Precautions:** Avoid if pregnant or breastfeeding.

11. **Oregano Oil Steam Inhalation**

- **Definition:** Inhalation of oregano oil-infused steam to clear nasal passages.

- **Ingredients:** Oregano essential oil, hot water.

- **How to Prepare:** Add a few drops of oregano oil to hot water, inhale steam.

- **How to Use:** Inhale steam for 5-10 minutes.

- **Dosage:** Use as needed.

- **Side Effects:** Inhalation may cause irritation in sensitive individuals.

- **Precautions:** Dilute oregano oil properly; avoid contact with eyes.

12. **Echinacea Tea**

- **Definition:** Echinacea tea helps boost the immune system and reduce mucus production.

- **Ingredients:** Dried echinacea leaves or roots, hot water.

- **How to Prepare:** Steep dried echinacea leaves or roots in hot water for 5-10 minutes.

- **How to Use:** Drink 1-2 cups daily.

- **Dosage:** 1-2 cups per day.

- **Side Effects:** May cause allergic reactions or gastrointestinal upset.

- **Precautions:** Avoid long-term use; not recommended for those with autoimmune disorders.

13. **Green Tea**

- **Definition:** Green tea is rich in antioxidants and helps support overall health.

- **Ingredients:** Green tea leaves, hot water.

- **How to Prepare:** Steep green tea leaves in hot water for 2-3 minutes.

- **How to Use:** Drink 1-3 cups daily.

- **Dosage:** 1-3 cups per day.

- **Side Effects:** May cause insomnia or stomach upset in some individuals.

- **Precautions:** Avoid excessive consumption, especially in sensitive individuals.

14. **Sage Tea**

- **Definition:** Sage tea helps relieve sore throat and reduce mucus production.

- **Ingredients:** Fresh or dried sage leaves, hot water.

- **How to Prepare:** Steep sage leaves in hot water for 5-10 minutes.

- **How to Use:** Drink 1-2 cups daily.

- **Dosage:** 1-2 cups per day.

- **Side Effects:** May cause allergic reactions or gastrointestinal upset.

- **Precautions:** Avoid if pregnant, breastfeeding, or have epilepsy.

15. **Rosemary Infusion**

- **Definition:** Rosemary infusion helps clear respiratory congestion and support immune health.

- **Ingredients:** Fresh or dried rosemary leaves, hot water.

- **How to Prepare:** Steep rosemary leaves in hot water for 5-10 minutes.

- **How to Use:** Drink 1-2 cups daily.

- **Dosage:** 1-2 cups per day.

- **Side Effects:** May cause allergic reactions or digestive upset.

- **Precautions:** Avoid if pregnant, breastfeeding, or have high blood pressure.

SOME HERBAL REMEDIS YOU SHOULD KNOW

Hydrangea:

Definition: Hydrangea, scientifically known as Hydrangea arborescens, is a flowering shrub native to North America. It has been used traditionally in herbal medicine for its potential diuretic and anti-inflammatory properties.

Ingredients: Hydrangea contains several bioactive compounds, including saponins, flavonoids, and glycosides. These compounds are believed to contribute to the herb's medicinal properties, including its potential as a diuretic, kidney tonic, and anti-inflammatory agent.

How to Prepare: Hydrangea root is typically prepared and consumed as an herbal tea or tincture. To make tea, dried hydrangea root is steeped in hot water for several minutes before being strained and consumed. Tinctures are prepared by steeping the root in alcohol or vinegar to extract its active compounds.

Dosage: The appropriate dosage of hydrangea can vary depending on factors such as age, health status, and the specific preparation being used. It's important to follow the recommended dosage on the product label or consult with a qualified herbalist or healthcare professional for personalized guidance.

How to Use: Hydrangea tea or tincture is typically taken orally. It's important to use hydrangea products as directed and to discontinue use if any adverse effects occur.

Side Effects: Hydrangea is generally considered safe for most people when used in moderate amounts. However, some individuals may experience digestive upset or allergic reactions. It may also interact with certain medications or have adverse effects in individuals with certain health conditions. It's important to use hydrangea under the guidance of a healthcare professional and to discontinue use if any adverse effects occur.

Irish Moss:

Definition: Irish Moss, scientifically known as Chondrus crispus, is a species of red algae or seaweed native to the Atlantic coastlines of Europe and North America. It has been used for centuries in traditional Irish and Scottish cuisine, as well as in herbal medicine.

Ingredients: Irish Moss is rich in various nutrients, including iodine, sulfur compounds, vitamins (such as vitamin A, vitamin K, and vitamin B12), minerals (including calcium, magnesium, potassium, and sodium), and polysaccharides (such as carrageenan). These nutrients are believed to contribute to the herb's potential health benefits.

How to Prepare: Irish Moss is typically prepared by soaking it in water to rehydrate and soften it before use. It can be added to soups, stews, smoothies, desserts, and other dishes as a thickening agent or nutritional supplement.

Dosage: The appropriate dosage of Irish Moss can vary depending on factors such as age, health status, and the specific preparation being used. It's important to follow recipes or guidelines for culinary use and to consult with a healthcare professional for guidance on using Irish Moss as a dietary supplement.

How to Use: Irish Moss can be used in culinary applications to add thickness and nutritional value to dishes. It can also be consumed as a dietary supplement in the form of capsules, powders, or extracts.

Side Effects: Irish Moss is generally considered safe for most people when consumed in moderate amounts as part of a balanced diet. However, some individuals may be allergic to seaweed or carrageenan, a compound found in Irish Moss that is used as a food additive. It's important to discontinue use if any adverse effects occur and to consult with a healthcare professional if you have any concerns.

Irish Sea Moss:

Definition: Irish Sea Moss is a term often used interchangeably with Irish Moss, referring to the same species of red algae, Chondrus crispus. It's harvested from the rocky shores of the Atlantic coastlines of Europe and North America.

Ingredients: Irish Sea Moss shares the same nutritional profile as Irish Moss, containing iodine, vitamins, minerals, and polysaccharides. It's valued for its potential health benefits, including supporting thyroid function, boosting immune health, and promoting digestion.

How to Prepare: Irish Sea Moss is prepared in the same way as Irish Moss, by soaking it in water to rehydrate and soften it before use. It can be used in culinary applications or consumed as a dietary supplement.

Dosage: The dosage of Irish Sea Moss depends on the form and intended use. As a dietary supplement, it's important to follow the recommended dosage on the product label or consult with a healthcare professional for personalized guidance.

How to Use: Irish Sea Moss can be used in various culinary applications, including soups, smoothies, desserts, and sauces. It can also be consumed as a dietary supplement in the form of capsules, powders, or extracts.

Side Effects: Similar to Irish Moss, Irish Sea Moss is generally considered safe for most people when consumed in moderate amounts. However, individuals with seaweed allergies or sensitivities to carrageenan should exercise caution. It's important to discontinue use if any adverse effects occur and to consult with a healthcare professional if you have any concerns.

Lymphalin:

Definition: Lymphalin is a herbal supplement formulated to support lymphatic system health. The lymphatic system plays a crucial role in immune function and waste removal in the body, and Lymphalin is designed to promote its proper function.

Ingredients: Lymphalin typically contains a blend of herbs and botanical extracts known for their traditional use in supporting lymphatic system health. Common ingredients may include cleavers, red clover, echinacea, burdock root, and calendula, among others.

How to Prepare: Lymphalin is usually available in capsule or liquid form. Capsules are taken orally with water, while liquid forms may be mixed with water or juice before consumption. It's important to follow the recommended dosage on the product label.

Dosage: The appropriate dosage of Lymphalin can vary depending on the specific product and individual needs. It's important to follow the recommended dosage on the product label or consult with a healthcare professional for personalized guidance.

How to Use: Lymphalin capsules are typically taken orally with water, while liquid forms may be mixed with water or juice before consumption. It's often recommended to take Lymphalin on an empty stomach for optimal absorption.

Side Effects: Lymphalin is generally considered safe for most people when used as directed. However, some individuals may experience mild side effects such as gastrointestinal discomfort or allergic reactions to certain ingredients. It's important to consult with a healthcare provider before starting any new supplement regimen, especially if you have underlying health conditions or are taking medications.

Manjakani:

Definition: Manjakani, also known as Quercus infectoria or oak gall, is a natural substance derived from the oak tree. It has been used for centuries in traditional medicine for its potential health benefits, particularly for women's health and vaginal tightening.

Ingredients: Manjakani contains various bioactive compounds, including tannins, flavonoids, and gallic acid. These compounds are believed to contribute to the herb's medicinal properties, including its potential as an astringent and antiseptic agent.

How to Prepare: Manjakani is typically available in powder, capsule, or liquid extract form. It can be taken orally or used topically depending on the intended use. For vaginal tightening, manjakani may be applied topically as a gel or inserted into the vagina in capsule form.

Dosage: The appropriate dosage of manjakani can vary depending on factors such as age, health status, and the specific preparation being used. It's important to follow the recommended dosage on the product label or consult with a qualified herbalist or healthcare professional for personalized guidance.

How to Use: Manjakani can be taken orally or used topically depending on the intended use. It's important to use manjakani products as directed and to discontinue use if any adverse effects occur.

Side Effects: Manjakani is generally considered safe for most people when used in moderate amounts. However, some individuals may experience allergic reactions or skin irritation when used topically. It's important to use manjakani under the guidance of a healthcare professional and to discontinue use if any adverse effects occur.

Red Clover:

Definition: Red clover, scientifically known as Trifolium pratense, is a flowering plant belonging to the legume family. It's native to Europe, Western Asia, and Northwest Africa but has been naturalized in many other regions. Red clover has been used in traditional medicine for various purposes, including its potential to support women's health and menopausal symptoms.

Ingredients: Red clover contains several bioactive compounds, including isoflavones (such as genistein and daidzein), flavonoids, and phytoestrogens. These compounds are believed to contribute to the herb's medicinal properties, including its potential as a hormone-balancing agent and its ability to support cardiovascular health.

How to Prepare: Red clover is typically prepared and consumed as an herbal tea or tincture. To make tea, dried red clover flowers are steeped in hot water for several minutes before being strained and consumed. Tinctures are prepared by steeping the flowers in alcohol or vinegar to extract their active compounds.

Dosage: The appropriate dosage of red clover can vary depending on factors such as age, health status, and the specific preparation being used. It's important to follow the recommended dosage on the product label or consult with a qualified herbalist or healthcare professional for personalized guidance.

How to Use: Red clover tea or tincture is typically taken orally. It's important to use red clover products as directed and to discontinue use if any adverse effects occur.

Side Effects: Red clover is generally considered safe for most people when used in moderate amounts. However, some individuals may experience allergic reactions or digestive upset. It may also interact with certain medications or have adverse effects in individuals with certain health conditions. It's important to use red clover under the guidance of a healthcare professional and to discontinue use if any adverse effects occur.

Red Raspberry:

Definition: Red raspberry, scientifically known as Rubus idaeus, is a species of raspberry native to Europe and northern Asia. It's widely cultivated for its delicious berries and has been used in traditional medicine for various purposes, including its potential to support women's health during pregnancy and childbirth.

Ingredients: Red raspberry contains several bioactive compounds, including flavonoids, ellagic acid, anthocyanins, and vitamin C. These compounds are believed to contribute to the herb's medicinal properties, including its potential as an antioxidant, anti-inflammatory, and uterine tonic.

How to Prepare: Red raspberry leaf is typically prepared and consumed as an herbal tea or infusion. To make tea, dried red raspberry leaves are steeped in hot water for several minutes before being strained and consumed.

Dosage: The appropriate dosage of red raspberry leaf can vary depending on factors such as age, health status, and the specific preparation being used. It's important to follow the recommended dosage on the product label or consult with a qualified herbalist or healthcare professional for personalized guidance.

How to Use: Red raspberry leaf tea is typically taken orally. It's often recommended for pregnant individuals in the later stages of pregnancy to support uterine health and prepare for childbirth. It's important to use red raspberry leaf products as directed and to discontinue use if any adverse effects occur.

Side Effects: Red raspberry leaf is generally considered safe for most people when used in moderate amounts. However, some individuals may experience allergic reactions or digestive upset. Pregnant individuals should consult with a healthcare professional before using red raspberry leaf, especially if they have any underlying health conditions or are taking medications. It's important to use red raspberry leaf under the guidance of a healthcare professional and to discontinue use if any adverse effects occur.

Rhubarb:

Definition: Rhubarb, scientifically known as Rheum rhabarbarum, is a perennial plant cultivated for its edible stalks. While primarily used in culinary applications, rhubarb has also been utilized in traditional medicine for its potential health benefits, particularly for digestive health.

Ingredients: Rhubarb stalks contain various bioactive compounds, including anthraquinones (such as emodin and rhein), fiber, vitamins (such as vitamin K), and minerals (including calcium and potassium). These compounds are believed to contribute to the herb's medicinal properties, including its potential as a laxative and digestive aid.

How to Prepare: Rhubarb stalks are typically cooked before consumption, as the raw stalks are very tart and can be unpleasant to eat. They are often used in pies, crisps, jams, sauces, and other desserts, as well as in savory dishes. Rhubarb can also be used to make compotes, jams, and preserves.

Dosage: There is no specific dosage for rhubarb in culinary applications, as it is used as a food rather than a medicinal herb. However, when used for its potential laxative effects, it's important to consume rhubarb in moderation to avoid gastrointestinal upset.

How to Use: Rhubarb stalks can be chopped and cooked in various dishes, including pies, sauces, and jams. It's important to remove and discard the leaves, as they contain toxic compounds. When using rhubarb for its potential laxative effects, it's typically consumed as part of a cooked dish or in the form of a rhubarb-based herbal remedy.

Side Effects: Rhubarb stalks are generally safe for most people when consumed in moderate amounts as part of a balanced diet.

However, excessive intake may lead to digestive upset or adverse effects due to the presence of oxalic acid, which can bind to calcium and form kidney stones in susceptible individuals. It's important to use rhubarb in moderation and to consult with a healthcare professional if you have any concerns or underlying health conditions.

Sarsaparilla:

Definition: Sarsaparilla refers to several species of plants belonging to the Smilax genus, including Smilax regelii and Smilax officinalis. It has been used historically in traditional medicine for its potential health benefits, particularly for its purported detoxifying and anti-inflammatory properties.

Ingredients: Sarsaparilla contains various bioactive compounds, including saponins (such as sarsaponin and smilagenin), flavonoids, phenolic acids, and sterols. These compounds are believed to contribute to the herb's medicinal properties, including its potential as a diuretic, blood purifier, and anti-inflammatory agent.

How to Prepare: Sarsaparilla root is typically prepared and consumed as an herbal tea, decoction, or tincture. To make tea, dried sarsaparilla root is steeped in hot water for several minutes before being strained and consumed. Decoctions involve boiling the root in water to extract its active compounds, while tinctures are prepared by steeping the root in alcohol or vinegar.

Dosage: The appropriate dosage of sarsaparilla can vary depending on factors such as age, health status, and the specific preparation being used. It's important to follow the recommended dosage on the product label or consult with a qualified herbalist or healthcare professional for personalized guidance.

How to Use: Sarsaparilla tea or tincture is typically taken orally. It's important to use sarsaparilla products as directed and to discontinue use if any adverse effects occur.

Side Effects: Sarsaparilla is generally considered safe for most people when used in moderate amounts. However, some individuals may experience allergic reactions or digestive upset. It may also interact with certain medications or have adverse effects in individuals with certain health conditions. It's important to use sarsaparilla under the guidance of a healthcare professional and to discontinue use if any adverse effects occur.

Tila:

Definition: Tila, also known as linden flower or lime blossom, refers to the flowers of the Tilia genus, primarily Tilia europaea and Tilia cordata. These trees are native to Europe, but they are also cultivated in other regions for their fragrant and medicinal flowers.

Ingredients: Tila flowers contain various bioactive compounds, including flavonoids, phenolic acids, and volatile oils. These compounds are believed to contribute to the herb's medicinal properties, including its potential as a mild sedative, anxiolytic, and anti-inflammatory agent.

How to Prepare: Tila flowers are typically prepared and consumed as an herbal tea or infusion. To make tea, dried tila flowers are steeped in hot water for several minutes before being strained and consumed.

Dosage: The appropriate dosage of tila can vary depending on factors such as age, health status, and the specific preparation being used. It's important to follow the recommended dosage on the product label or consult with a qualified herbalist or healthcare professional for personalized guidance.

How to Use: Tila tea is typically taken orally. It's often consumed in the evening as a calming bedtime beverage or during times of stress or anxiety. It's important to use tila products as directed and to discontinue use if any adverse effects occur.

Side Effects: Tila is generally considered safe for most people when used in moderate amounts. However, some individuals may experience allergic reactions or digestive upset. It may also interact with certain medications or have adverse effects in individuals with certain health conditions. It's important to use tila under the guidance of a healthcare professional and to discontinue use if any adverse effects occur.

Valerian:

Definition: Valerian, scientifically known as Valeriana officinalis, is a perennial flowering plant native to Europe and Asia. It has been used for centuries in traditional medicine for its potential calming and sedative effects.

Ingredients: Valerian root contains several bioactive compounds, including valerenic acid, valepotriates, and volatile oils. These compounds are believed to contribute to the herb's medicinal properties, including its potential as a sedative, anxiolytic, and sleep aid.

How to Prepare: Valerian root is typically prepared and consumed as an herbal tea, tincture, or capsule. To make tea, dried valerian root is steeped in hot water for several minutes before being strained and consumed. Tinctures are prepared by steeping the root in alcohol or vinegar to extract its active compounds.

Dosage: The appropriate dosage of valerian can vary depending on factors such as age, health status, and the specific preparation being used. It's important to follow the recommended dosage on the product label or consult with a qualified herbalist or healthcare professional for personalized guidance.

How to Use: Valerian tea, tincture, or capsules are typically taken orally. It's often consumed in the evening as a sleep aid or during times of stress or anxiety. It's important to use valerian products as directed and to discontinue use if any adverse effects occur.

Side Effects: Valerian is generally considered safe for most people when used in moderate amounts. However, some individuals may experience mild side effects such as drowsiness, headache, or gastrointestinal upset. It may also interact with certain medications or have adverse effects in individuals with certain health conditions. It's important to use valerian under the guidance of a healthcare professional and to discontinue use if any adverse effects occur.

Wild Cherry Bark:

Definition: Wild cherry bark, scientifically known as Prunus serotina, is the bark obtained from the black cherry tree native to North America. It has been used traditionally in Native American and folk medicine for its potential health benefits, particularly for respiratory and digestive issues.

Ingredients: Wild cherry bark contains various bioactive compounds, including cyanogenic glycosides (such as prunasin and amygdalin), flavonoids, and phenolic acids. These compounds are believed to contribute to the herb's medicinal properties, including its potential as an expectorant, cough suppressant, and mild sedative.

How to Prepare: Wild cherry bark is typically prepared and consumed as an herbal tea, decoction, or syrup. To make tea, dried wild cherry bark is steeped in hot water for several minutes before being strained and consumed. Decoctions involve boiling the bark in water to extract its active compounds, while syrups are made by simmering the bark with sugar or honey to create a thick, sweet liquid.

Dosage: The appropriate dosage of wild cherry bark can vary depending on factors such as age, health status, and the specific preparation being used. It's important to follow the recommended dosage on the product label or consult with a qualified herbalist or healthcare professional for personalized guidance.

How to Use: Wild cherry bark tea, decoction, or syrup is typically taken orally. It's often consumed to soothe coughs, sore throats, and other respiratory symptoms. It's important to use wild cherry bark products as directed and to discontinue use if any adverse effects occur.

Side Effects: Wild cherry bark is generally considered safe for most people when used in moderate amounts. However, it contains cyanogenic glycosides, which can release cyanide in the body when metabolized. While the risk of cyanide poisoning from consuming wild cherry bark is low when used appropriately, excessive intake or prolonged use may lead to adverse effects. It's important to use wild cherry bark under the guidance of a healthcare professional and to discontinue use if any adverse effects occur.

Yellowdock:

Definition: Yellowdock, scientifically known as Rumex crispus, is a perennial flowering plant native to Europe and western Asia but is also found in North America. It has a long history of use in traditional medicine, particularly among Indigenous peoples, for its potential health benefits.

Ingredients: Yellowdock root contains various bioactive compounds, including anthraquinone glycosides (such as emodin and chrysophanol), tannins, and vitamins (including vitamin A and vitamin C). These compounds are believed to contribute to the herb's medicinal properties, including its potential as a laxative, blood cleanser, and liver tonic.

How to Prepare: Yellowdock root is typically prepared and consumed as an herbal tea, tincture, or capsule. To make tea, dried yellowdock root is steeped in hot water for several minutes before being strained and consumed. Tinctures are prepared by steeping the root in alcohol or vinegar to extract its active compounds.

Dosage: The appropriate dosage of yellowdock can vary depending on factors such as age, health status, and the specific preparation being used. It's important to follow the recommended dosage on the product label or consult with a qualified herbalist or healthcare professional for personalized guidance.

How to Use: Yellowdock tea, tincture, or capsules are typically taken orally. It's often consumed to support digestion, promote bowel regularity, and cleanse the blood. It's important to use yellowdock products as directed and to discontinue use if any adverse effects occur.

Side Effects: Yellowdock is generally considered safe for most people when used in moderate amounts. However, some individuals may experience mild side effects such as gastrointestinal upset or allergic reactions. It may also interact with certain medications or have adverse effects in individuals with certain health conditions. It's important to use yellowdock under the guidance of a healthcare professional and to discontinue use if any adverse effects occur.

Yellowdock Root:

Definition: Yellowdock root, scientifically known as Rumex crispus, is the root of a perennial flowering plant native to Europe and western Asia, also found in North America. It has a long history of use in traditional medicine, particularly among Indigenous peoples, for its potential health benefits.

Ingredients: Yellowdock root contains various bioactive compounds, including anthraquinone glycosides (such as emodin and chrysophanol), tannins, and vitamins (including vitamin A and vitamin C). These compounds are believed to contribute to the herb's medicinal properties, including its potential as a laxative, blood cleanser, and liver tonic.

How to Prepare: Yellowdock root is typically prepared and consumed as an herbal tea, tincture, or capsule. To make tea, dried yellowdock root is steeped in hot water for several minutes before being strained and consumed. Tinctures are prepared by steeping the root in alcohol or vinegar to extract its active compounds.

Dosage: The appropriate dosage of yellowdock root can vary depending on factors such as age, health status, and the specific preparation being used. It's important to follow the recommended dosage on the product label or consult with a qualified herbalist or healthcare professional for personalized guidance.

How to Use: Yellowdock root tea, tincture, or capsules are typically taken orally. It's often consumed to support digestion, promote bowel regularity, and cleanse the blood. It's important to use yellowdock root products as directed and to discontinue use if any adverse effects occur.

Side Effects: Yellowdock root is generally considered safe for most people when used in moderate amounts. However, some individuals may experience mild side effects such as gastrointestinal upset or allergic reactions. It may also interact with certain medications or have adverse effects in individuals with certain health conditions. It's important to use yellowdock root under the guidance of a healthcare professional and to discontinue use if any adverse effects occur.

Agrimony:

Definition: Agrimony, scientifically known as Agrimonia eupatoria, is a perennial herbaceous plant native to Europe, Asia, and North America. It has a long history of use in traditional medicine, particularly in European folk medicine, for its potential health benefits.

Ingredients: Agrimony contains various bioactive compounds, including tannins, flavonoids, phenolic acids, and volatile oils. These compounds are believed to contribute to the herb's medicinal properties, including its potential as an astringent, anti-inflammatory, and digestive aid.

How to Prepare: Agrimony is typically prepared and consumed as an herbal tea, tincture, or poultice. To make tea, dried agrimony leaves and flowers are steeped in hot water for several minutes before being strained and consumed. Tinctures are prepared by steeping the herb in alcohol or vinegar to extract its active compounds.

Dosage: The appropriate dosage of agrimony can vary depending on factors such as age, health status, and the specific preparation being used. It's important to follow the recommended dosage on the product label or consult with a qualified herbalist or healthcare professional for personalized guidance.

How to Use: Agrimony tea, tincture, or poultice is typically taken orally or applied topically. It's often consumed to soothe gastrointestinal issues, such as indigestion and diarrhea, or used externally to treat skin conditions.

Side Effects: Agrimony is generally considered safe for most people when used in moderate amounts. However, some individuals may experience allergic reactions or gastrointestinal upset. It may also interact with certain medications or have adverse effects in individuals with certain health conditions. It's important to use agrimony under the guidance of a healthcare professional and to discontinue use if any adverse effects occur.

Alfalfa:

Definition: Alfalfa, scientifically known as Medicago sativa, is a flowering plant in the pea family native to Asia but cultivated worldwide. It's primarily grown as fodder for livestock, but it has also been used in traditional medicine for its potential health benefits.

Ingredients: Alfalfa contains various bioactive compounds, including vitamins (such as vitamin A, vitamin C, and vitamin K), minerals (including calcium, magnesium, and potassium), amino acids, and phytoestrogens. These compounds are believed to contribute to the herb's medicinal properties, including its potential as a nutritive tonic, diuretic, and hormone balancer.

How to Prepare: Alfalfa is typically consumed as sprouts, herbal tea, or in supplement form (such as capsules or tablets). To make tea, dried alfalfa leaves are steeped in hot water for several minutes before being strained and consumed.

Dosage: The appropriate dosage of alfalfa can vary depending on factors such as age, health status, and the specific preparation being used. It's important to follow the recommended dosage on the product label or consult with a qualified herbalist or healthcare professional for personalized guidance.

How to Use: Alfalfa sprouts, tea, or supplements are typically taken orally. It's often consumed as a dietary supplement to support overall health and well-being, as well as to promote kidney health and hormone balance.

Side Effects: Alfalfa is generally considered safe for most people when consumed in moderate amounts. However, some individuals may experience allergic reactions or digestive upset. It may also interact with certain medications or have adverse effects in individuals with certain health conditions, such as autoimmune diseases or hormone-sensitive conditions. Pregnant or breastfeeding individuals should consult with a healthcare professional before using alfalfa supplements. It's important to use alfalfa under the guidance of a healthcare professional and to discontinue use if any adverse effects occur.

Ashwagandha:

Definition: Ashwagandha, scientifically known as Withaniasomnifera, is a small shrub native to India, the Middle East, and parts of Africa. It has a long history of use in Ayurvedic medicine for its potential health benefits, particularly for its adaptogenic properties.

Ingredients: Ashwagandha root contains various bioactive compounds, including alkaloids (such as withanolides), steroidal lactones, and flavonoids. These compounds are believed to contribute to the herb's medicinal properties, including its potential as an adaptogen, anti-inflammatory, and immune-modulating agent.

How to Prepare: Ashwagandha is typically consumed as a powdered root, herbal tea, tincture, or in supplement form (such as capsules or tablets). To make tea, dried ashwagandha root is steeped in hot water for several minutes before being strained and consumed.

Dosage: The appropriate dosage of ashwagandha can vary depending on factors such as age, health status, and the specific preparation being used. It's important to follow the recommended dosage on the product label or consult with a qualified herbalist or healthcare professional for personalized guidance.

How to Use: Ashwagandha powder, tea, tincture, or supplements are typically taken orally. It's often consumed to support stress management, promote relaxation, and boost overall vitality and well-being.

Side Effects: Ashwagandha is generally considered safe for most people when used in moderate amounts. However, some individuals may experience mild side effects such as gastrointestinal upset or drowsiness. It may also interact with certain medications or have adverse effects in individuals with certain health conditions, such as autoimmune diseases or thyroid disorders. Pregnant or breastfeeding individuals should consult with a healthcare professional before using ashwagandha supplements. It's important to use ashwagandha under the guidance of a healthcare professional and to discontinue use if any adverse effects occur.

Black Cohosh:

Definition: Black cohosh, scientifically known as Actaea racemosa (formerly Cimicifuga racemosa), is a perennial herb native to North America. It has a long history of use in traditional Native American medicine and later in folk medicine for its potential health benefits, particularly for women's health.

Ingredients: Black cohosh root contains various bioactive compounds, including triterpene glycosides (such as actein and cimicifugoside), phenolic acids, and flavonoids. These compounds are believed to contribute to the herb's medicinal properties, including its potential as a hormone-balancing agent and its ability to relieve menopausal symptoms.

How to Prepare: Black cohosh is typically consumed as a powdered root, herbal tea, tincture, or in supplement form (such as capsules or tablets). To make tea, dried black cohosh root is steeped in hot water for several minutes before being strained and consumed.

Dosage: The appropriate dosage of black cohosh can vary depending on factors such as age, health status, and the specific preparation being used. It's important to follow the recommended dosage on the product label or consult with a qualified herbalist or healthcare professional for personalized guidance.

How to Use: Black cohosh powder, tea, tincture, or supplements are typically taken orally. It's often used by women to support hormonal balance, relieve menopausal symptoms such as hot flashes and night sweats, and promote overall well-being.

Side Effects: Black cohosh is generally considered safe for most people when used in moderate amounts. However, some individuals may experience mild side effects such as gastrointestinal upset or allergic reactions. It may also interact with certain medications or have adverse effects in individuals with certain health conditions, such as liver disease or hormone-sensitive conditions. Pregnant or breastfeeding individuals should consult with a healthcare professional before using black cohosh supplements. It's important to use black cohosh under the guidance of a healthcare professional and to discontinue use if any adverse effects occur.

Chickweed:

Definition: Chickweed, scientifically known as Stellaria media, is an annual herbaceous plant native to Europe but naturalized in many other parts of the world. It's often considered a common weed but has been used historically in traditional medicine for its potential health benefits.

Ingredients: Chickweed contains various bioactive compounds, including flavonoids, saponins, mucilage, and vitamins (such as vitamin C). These compounds are believed to contribute to the herb's medicinal properties, including its potential as a demulcent, anti-inflammatory, and mild diuretic.

How to Prepare: Chickweed is typically consumed as an herbal tea, infusion, or in fresh salads. To make tea, dried chickweed leaves and flowers are steeped in hot water for several minutes before being strained and consumed. It can also be used topically as a poultice or infused oil for skin conditions.

Dosage: The appropriate dosage of chickweed can vary depending on factors such as age, health status, and the specific preparation being used. It's important to follow the recommended dosage on the product label or consult with a qualified herbalist or healthcare professional for personalized guidance.

How to Use: Chickweed tea, infusion, or fresh leaves are typically taken orally. It's often used to soothe inflammation, support digestion, and promote overall well-being. Topically, chickweed can be applied to the skin to alleviate itching, irritation, or minor wounds.

Side Effects: Chickweed is generally considered safe for most people when consumed in moderate amounts. However, some individuals may experience allergic reactions or gastrointestinal upset. It may also interact with certain medications or have adverse effects in individuals with certain health conditions. Pregnant or breastfeeding individuals should consult with a healthcare professional before using chickweed supplements. It's important to use chickweed under the guidance of a healthcare professional and to discontinue use if any adverse effects occur.

Blessed Thistle:

Definition: Blessed thistle, scientifically known as Cnicusbenedictus, is an annual or biennial herb native to the Mediterranean region but also found in other parts of Europe, Asia, and North Africa. It has been used historically in traditional medicine for its potential health benefits, particularly for digestive and liver health.

Ingredients: Blessed thistle contains various bioactive compounds, including sesquiterpene lactones (such as cnicin), flavonoids, tannins, and essential oils. These compounds are believed to contribute to the herb's medicinal properties, including its potential as a digestive tonic, appetite stimulant, and liver tonic.

How to Prepare: Blessed thistle is typically consumed as an herbal tea, tincture, or in supplement form (such as capsules or tablets). To make tea, dried blessed thistle leaves and flowers are steeped in hot water for several minutes before being strained and consumed.

Dosage: The appropriate dosage of blessed thistle can vary depending on factors such as age, health status, and the specific preparation being used. It's important to follow the recommended dosage on the product label or consult with a qualified herbalist or healthcare professional for personalized guidance.

How to Use: Blessed thistle tea, tincture, or supplements are typically taken orally. It's often used to support digestion, stimulate appetite, and promote liver health.

Side Effects: Blessed thistle is generally considered safe for most people when used in moderate amounts. However, some individuals may experience mild side effects such as gastrointestinal upset or allergic reactions. It may also interact with certain medications or have adverse effects in individuals with certain health conditions, such as hormone-sensitive conditions or bleeding disorders. Pregnant or breastfeeding individuals should consult with a healthcare professional before using blessed thistle supplements. It's important to use blessed thistle under the guidance of a healthcare professional and to discontinue use if any adverse effects occur.

Cat's Claw:

Definition: Cat's claw, scientifically known as Uncaria tomentosa, is a woody vine native to the Amazon rainforest and other parts of Central and South America. It has been used for centuries in traditional medicine by indigenous peoples for its potential health benefits.

Ingredients: Cat's claw contains various bioactive compounds, including alkaloids (such as oxindole alkaloids and quinovic acid glycosides), polyphenols, and other phytochemicals. These compounds are believed to contribute to the herb's medicinal properties, including its potential as an immune enhancer, anti-inflammatory, and antioxidant.

How to Prepare: Cat's claw is typically consumed as an herbal tea, tincture, or in supplement form (such as capsules or tablets). To make tea, dried cat's claw bark or leaves are steeped in hot water for several minutes before being strained and consumed.

Dosage: The appropriate dosage of cat's claw can vary depending on factors such as age, health status, and the specific preparation being used. It's important to follow the recommended dosage on the product label or consult with a qualified herbalist or healthcare professional for personalized guidance.

How to Use: Cat's claw tea, tincture, or supplements are typically taken orally. It's often used to support immune function, reduce inflammation, and promote overall well-being.

Side Effects: Cat's claw is generally considered safe for most people when used in moderate amounts. However, some individuals may experience mild side effects such as gastrointestinal upset or allergic reactions. It may also interact with certain medications or have adverse effects in individuals with certain health conditions, such as autoimmune diseases or bleeding disorders. Pregnant or breastfeeding individuals should consult with a healthcare professional before using cat's claw supplements. It's important to use cat's claw under the guidance of a healthcare professional and to discontinue use if any adverse effects occur.

Astragalus:

Definition: Astragalus, scientifically known as Astragalus membranaceus, is a flowering plant native to China and Mongolia but also found in other parts of Asia. It has been used for centuries in traditional Chinese medicine for its potential health benefits, particularly for its immune-enhancing properties.

Ingredients: Astragalus root contains various bioactive compounds, including polysaccharides, saponins (such as astragalosides), flavonoids, and amino acids. These compounds are believed to contribute to the herb's medicinal properties, including its potential as an adaptogen, immunomodulator, and anti-inflammatory agent.

How to Prepare: Astragalus is typically consumed as a powdered root, herbal tea, tincture, or in supplement form (such as capsules or tablets). To make tea, dried astragalus root slices are simmered in water for several minutes before being strained and consumed.

Dosage: The appropriate dosage of astragalus can vary depending on factors such as age, health status, and the specific preparation being used. It's important to follow the recommended dosage on the product label or consult with a qualified herbalist or healthcare professional for personalized guidance.

How to Use: Astragalus powder, tea, tincture, or supplements are typically taken orally. It's often consumed to support immune function, promote vitality, and enhance overall well-being.

Side Effects: Astragalus is generally considered safe for most people when used in moderate amounts. However, some individuals may experience mild side effects such as gastrointestinal upset or allergic reactions. It may also interact with certain medications or have adverse effects in individuals with certain health conditions, such as autoimmune diseases or diabetes. Pregnant or breastfeeding individuals should consult with a healthcare professional before using astragalus supplements. It's important to use astragalus under the guidance of a healthcare professional and to discontinue use if any adverse effects occur.

THE END